Dirty Talk

Enhance The Intimacy And Romantic Connection Within
Your Relationship By Engaging In Rousing Activities,
Utilizing Provocative Inquiries, And Indulging In Explicit
Communication

(Exemplifying The Paragon Of Amorous Proficiency)

Freddie Lewis

TABLE OF CONTENT

What Does The Term 'Dirty Talk' Denote, And Can It Yield Successful Outcomes For You?

Erotic discourse involves the deliberate utilization of verbal expressions to evoke vivid and explicit mental imagery, with the aim of heightening sexual arousal. This process occurs at a chemical and neurological level that the human body cannot refute. Engaging in provocative communication with your partner promotes an intensified state of longing and passion.

In my personal experience, engaging in risqué conversation holds a profound allure, evoking feelings of sensuality and anticipation, particularly when the circumstances are conducive. When the synchronization of my mind and body manifests in harmonious resonance. When my primal urges and yearnings supersede my apprehensions and vulnerabilities dissipate.

Conversing in a provocative manner constitutes the articulate manifestation of my profound desires, inclinations, requirements, and imaginings. Engaging in explicit or risqué conversation is a realm I venture into only in moments of utmost relaxation, arousal, and willingness to intimately connect with another individual. The sensation of their touch, their fragrance, even the mere thought of their presence elicits impulsive verbal expressions within my consciousness.

Engaging in explicit communication provides an opportunity to tap into one's innate instincts, a desire solely focused on experiencing gratification. It facilitates the act of immersing oneself fully in the present moment. The convergence of your thoughts and physical being gives rise to a sudden outpouring of words. The unbridled, primal desires within you collide with a symphony of seductive and alluring language.

This literature aims to provide a comprehensive resource for women wishing to embark upon the extensive realm of erotic conversation. I derive immense pleasure from observing the heightened state of arousal experienced by my partner when engaging in explicit communication during intimate moments. I am highly aroused by the profound focus in his gaze and the evident surge of desire within him, triggered by the mere sound of my voice. I derive immense pleasure from his articulate and sensual responses conveyed in his alluring and husky tonality. It elicits a heightened state of arousal within me, leading to a corresponding level of intimacy and desire from my partner. Engaging in explicit communication has significantly enhanced my sexual experiences, and I am confident that it has the potential to do the same for you.

Good Bye Boring Sex

There is a general aversion towards engaging in unsatisfying sexual encounters. If you are perusing this literary work, it is representative of your understanding as a woman of the significance of cultivating a fulfilling and satisfying sexual experience. Satisfactory sexual experiences may be acceptable, but extraordinary sexual encounters have the ability to profoundly alter one's life.

When the intimate aspect of a relationship becomes monotonous, it can give rise to tension and dissension. You may begin to question whether your partner's interest is waning or whether they no longer perceive you as desirable. He might be harboring identical queries concerning your situation.

It is unjust for any individual to endure a relationship wherein they experience sexual dissatisfaction. Whether you and your partner have been in a long-term committed relationship and desire to add excitement, or if you are actively exploring various romantic prospects, engaging in intimate verbal exchanges can heighten passion within the confines of the bedroom and extend into other aspects of your relationship.

Engaging in erotic dialogue has the potential to unlock unexplored realms of sexual potential. When engaging in intimate conversation while in bed, you have the opportunity to explore and express your most profound desires and fantasies. Engaging in sensual dialogue serves as a stimulating catalyst, intensifying the connection within your partnership and unveiling opportunities where you can freely explore your uninhibited nature.

Another advantage is that the majority of individuals of the male gender aspire to excel in their abilities as intimate partners; however, they may lack the necessary knowledge or know-how to accomplish this. Males tend to appreciate it when you communicate their preference or pleasure. They derive pleasure from listening to your desires related to their actions within an intimate setting. Men also greatly appreciate hearing about your intentions towards them.

With the passage of time, the intensity of physical attraction may diminish. As time progresses, we experience the natural progression of aging, accompanied by changes in our physical appearance and body contours. Explicit communication delves into cognitive faculties, serving as an influential catalyst for arousal within our corporeal selves. By imbuing your male partner's thoughts with sensual concepts and imagery, you will awaken his most profound yearnings. He will experience an overwhelming surge of intense desire upon contemplating your physical presence and when hearing the sound of your voice.

The Advantages of Erotic Communication

Engaging in explicit dialogue can aid in broadening one's sphere of personal ease and familiarity.

Engaging in erotic conversation facilitates the exploration of novel fantasies and concepts.

Engaging in explicit conversation enhances the establishment of trust and facilitates effective communication.

Dirty talk enhances foreplay.

Engaging in explicit conversation can provide valuable insights into one's own personal nature.

Engaging in explicit conversation can facilitate the discovery of novel aspects about one's partner.

Engaging in explicit conversation enhances the intensity of intimate encounters.

Engaging in explicit communication has the potential to arouse your partner, regardless of the physical proximity between you.

8

Incorporate One's Personal Ethics And Principles

It is of utmost importance to address your personal beliefs and principles when engaging in conversations about sex and sexuality with your child.

It is imperative to initially take into account your personal values and principles when discussing avian and insect reproductive matters with your child.

Rest assured that employing this approach will undoubtedly enhance your child's understanding of the situation.

It is essential to bear in mind that parents wield a substantial influence in shaping their children's lives. Consequently, it becomes imperative to exert a positive effect on parents, guiding them toward making sound decisions so that their children will be empowered to make optimal choices.

Effectively and Appropriately Communicating with Your Child about Human Sexuality

To initiate your discourse, it is crucial to ensure an adequate inclusion of scholarly sources and to articulate your own ethical principles and values. A parent possessing robust moral compass and deeply ingrained principles can significantly contribute to their child's management of matters pertaining to sex and sexuality.

Defeat your embarrassment

It is comprehensible if the mention of terms such as penis and vagina initially elicits discomfort.

It is recommended that you practice reciting these phrases discreetly on several occasions until you feel sufficiently at ease to discuss them with your child in a composed manner, thereby resolving your feelings of awkwardness.

One may find that engaging in this practice can result in a heightened sense of comfort and tranquility when conversing with one's child about matters pertaining to sexuality. This is considered to be one of the most effective approaches for promptly alleviating your embarrassment.

Arrange for the establishment of ongoing and interactive dialogues with your child.

According to experts, it is of utmost importance to provide your child with education regarding sex and sexuality, particularly during their early years.

Moreover, as children mature, it is imperative that you persist in imparting knowledge concerning this matter.

Your child will encounter matters pertaining to sex and sexuality throughout their lifetime, and it remains challenging to cover all aspects comprehensively within a single conversation.

Once you have successfully facilitated an open dialogue and established effective communication with your young individual, enable the expression of factual information and encourage the natural progression of discussing varying perspectives. Avail oneself of the opportunities provided for the acquisition of knowledge.

When one is accompanied by their child and comes across a pregnant woman or becomes aware of sexual events through media channels, as an illustration.

These educational instances possess the capability of facilitating smooth transitions and evolving into discussions concerning sexual predicaments. Consequently, educational opportunities will aid you in facilitating discussions relating to sexual matters, especially as your child approaches the age of adulthood.

Provide your child with comprehensive information.

Acquiring comprehensive knowledge and accurate details about sexual matters is an essential ethical principle and value that every parent ought to possess.

In recent years, the dissemination of inclusive sexual education material has become increasingly accessible through online platforms. Additionally, it is possible to provide your child with books that are suitable for their age to peruse.

If your child poses a question for which you do not possess the answer, it is appropriate to inform them that you will conduct research and subsequently provide them with a response.

Foresee the Progression of the Developmental Phase

It is advisable to refrain from discussing nocturnal emissions and menstruation with your child after they have experienced these phenomena for a few months. Prior to your child reaching adolescence, the initial subject you should discuss

The topic that they discuss pertains to sexual encounters and the various aspects of adolescence.

By implementing this approach, you will observe a reduction in your child's preoccupation with the changes occurring in their physique.

Please Don\\\'t Lecture.

Refrain from delivering lectures, as contemporary children tend to have minimal receptiveness towards this approach. It is highly advisable to furnish ample information and data, and engage in comprehensive deliberations pertaining to the subject matter. As a responsible parent, it is vital that you equip your child with appropriate resources and knowledge to enable them to make informed decisions regarding their sexual preferences and actions. Discussions and deliberations will indisputably prove more beneficial to your young one than monotonous lectures. You can have confidence that your adolescent will be attentive to you and regard your words with importance.

Educate Them on the Risks and Rewards of Sexual Activity

As per research findings, sexuality should not be considered an adverse aspect of human existence, and therefore, there is no rational basis for apprehension or fear related to it. Conversely, certain individuals hold the viewpoint that sexual activity carries inherent risks.

Sexuality is a innate facet of human existence, imparting an inherent beauty, and thus, it is imperative that your child possesses accurate knowledge and comprehensive comprehension of this realm.

Furthermore, they possess the entitlement to grasp the concepts of sexuality and sex, as well as acquire the necessary skills to effectively navigate and embrace these roles within the context of their existence.

Engaging in conversations with your child regarding relationships and intimacy will greatly contribute to their comprehensive understanding of this subject matter. As a responsible guardian, it is crucial that you promptly initiate communication with them, ensuring that your child develops a comprehensive understanding of human sexuality.

Use of emojis

Many young women hold varying perspectives on this matter. I would employ emojis in a moderate fashion. It is preferable to avoid adopting a demeanor reminiscent of a middle school girl engaging in communication with a romantic interest. Please refrain from using a excessive amount of 10 emojis when attempting to convey your message. On average, I employ a limited range of four to five distinct emojis.

Furthermore, refrain from utilizing them excessively in each and every textual communication. Employ a rotating approach, utilizing them interchangeably after every series of three to four texts.

Here are several options that you may consider utilizing:

*Smiley face

*Kissy face

*Cucumber

*Purple devil

The optimal locations and moments for engaging in sexting activities

An integral aspect of becoming proficient in engaging in intimate electronic communication (if one may use such terminology, for it appears to be a neologism) lies in discerning the most opportune moments and settings to engage in said activity with one's significant other.

Clearly, it would be inappropriate to engage in sexting while he is attending a crucial business meeting, spending time with his mother, or driving amidst traffic (refrain from sexting while operating a vehicle!).

Let us discuss the preferred location and time for engaging in intimate messaging.

Early in the morning

For couples who do not cohabitate, engaging in early morning text exchanges of an intimate nature can cultivate a heightened sense of excitement and anticipation in anticipation of future rendezvous.

Deliver a provocative message to him at the start of the day. Inform him that I had a dream involving him during the previous evening. I am completely soaked this morning. This will guarantee that he will remain constantly preoccupied with thoughts of you throughout the day.

If you are feeling particularly mischievous, consider sending him an image of your damp undergarments. Alternatively, it would be preferable for you to directly convey your message to him through a video recording, while delicately touching your undergarments with your fingertips.

If he is exposed to such imagery early in the morning, he will experience heightened arousal for the entirety of the day. Establishing a positive atmosphere in the morning can noticeably enhance the overall quality of anyone's day.

Amidst his midday reprieve

Doesn't everyone have a designated interval for lunch? Retrieve his agenda and discreetly transmit a provocative message during his midday break. He will be fully engaged in contemplating your presence, which aligns precisely with your desires.

Presented here is an enticing activity to engage in with your partner. Inform him that you are experiencing a strong sexual desire for his genitals. Please inform him to proceed to the restroom and capture an image of his genitalia for your reference. That will undoubtedly stimulate his cognitive processes!

If his workplace is in close proximity to our residence, perhaps consider messaging him with a statement like "On one of these occasions, I look forward to the opportunity of having you return home during your break to dine together."

Together in public

Engaging in explicit messaging with him in a public setting is inappropriate. Observe the expression of delight on his countenance as he peruses the suggestive message you sent him while in a public dining establishment or café.

The primary concept underlying the notion of engaging in public sexting is rooted in the notion that engaging in sexual activity in public spaces is forbidden, thus stimulating one's mind with a plethora of unfulfilled desires and stimulating thoughts. Sow those seeds and upon your return, he will anxiously desire to remove your undergarments.

Presented below are a selection of suitable public locations to engage in explicit digital communication with him:

Diners who wish to enhance their romantic dining experience may discreetly visit the restroom and capture intimate photographs to share with their partner. Please ensure that you spend a sufficient amount of time in the bathroom, so as to arouse curiosity as to your activities.

Coffee: In the interim as you queue for your coffee or make a purchase at the store, dispatch a message or item to his attention. It will serve as a pastime and stimulate his sexual desire.

Shopping: If you are engaging in a joint shopping excursion, consider visiting Victoria's Secret and partaking in the experience of trying on their clothing items. Capture a few photographs and observe the resulting outcomes.

When he\\\'s flying

Is it of concern to you that other women may engage in flirtatious behavior with your partner during their business travels? Ensure that you consistently occupy his thoughts through the exchange of provocative text messages.

Deliver him flirtatious messages while he is at the airport. Expressing a sentiment such as "I wish you were here to give me a cavity search" is inappropriate and offensive in formal communication. However, if you are seeking to convey a desire for the person's presence and assistance in a professional context, you could rephrase it as follows: "I would greatly appreciate your presence and thorough examination in order to ensure compliance with all necessary procedures and requirements."

Perhaps consider presenting him with a photograph depicting yourself adorned in a robe, coupled with articulate expressions detailing the profound necessity for the act of being thoroughly examined. Bestow upon him a genuine awareness of the extent to which he is absent from such an experience.

Currently, the majority of aircrafts are equipped with wireless internet connectivity. Please instruct him to acquire the in-flight wifi service (certain flights may offer complimentary wifi).

Presently, you have effectively confined him at an altitude of 10,000 feet for an extensive duration. It would be advisable to transmit improper textual content, visual media, and audio recordings to him. He will be writhing uncomfortably in his chair. Indeed, it is possible that upon arrival, he may completely abandon the planned journey and choose to return home by air.

Engaging in digital intimacy while he is airborne or absent from his place of residence is consistently quite enjoyable.

I thoroughly enjoy engaging in this activity with my partner. It consistently instills within him a desire to expedite his return to his place of residence.

When he is socializing with his male friends

Is he frequently engaging in social activities with his male friends? Ensure that he feels remorse for opting to spend time with his companions.

Send him a suggestive text message while he is socializing with his friends at the bar or attending a sports event. Ensure that he gains a comprehensive understanding of what he is forfeiting.

I am experiencing strong sexual arousal. I desire the presence of a companion to engage in intimate activities. If he is attending a sporting event, consider adorning a jersey representing a player he greatly admires and send him a tastefully enticing photograph. You will occupy his thoughts throughout the duration!

Kindly forward an image or video capturing your interaction with your feline companion, specifically showcasing the act performed through your undergarments. This combination will prompt him to immediately return home in haste. His acquaintances will struggle to comprehend the reason behind his haste to depart.

Chapter 7:

Conquer the Embarrassment of Indecent
Language

I am uncertain if you feel the same way,
but expressing explicit language is
particularly challenging, and one must
overcome this obstacle. Hey, I
understand. The preliminary encounter
may be somewhat uncomfortable. I must
be sincere with you. You may possess an
multitude of diverse ideas within your
mind. Might there be a chance that he
will reach the inference that I possess a
lack of intelligence? Is he under the
impression that I am engaged in the
profession of prostitution? Does it have
the potential to meet his satisfaction?
This should bring a sense of comfort, yet
it only results in an uncomfortable
experience."

Please be aware that a significant
number of men greatly appreciate and
are positively inclined towards engaging

in explicit and provocative conversations. Why? As a result of their inclination, they often ponder in a clandestine manner about whether you reciprocate their desired affection. Would you be interested in furthering your knowledge? As he is cognizant of your willingness to venture into the realm of prohibition solely for his sake, once you unleash your mischievous inclinations, he will ardently yearn for an escalation of such indulgence. Furthermore, he is immensely pleased by the fact that he has facilitated your arrival at that location.

Please be aware that it is entirely appropriate to openly communicate your sexual desires and thoughts. Engaging in explicit language is not inherently indecent. It is inherently customary, and although it may not arise immediately, it will ultimately transpire. Relinquish control over your vocal expressions and grant yourself the authority to confront him according to your long-held desires.

Would you like me to reveal a confidential piece of information to you? It is unlikely that the remaining content of the book will require your attention, as you can conveniently advance to the exemplifications provided, granted that you thoroughly comprehend the forthcoming information. Seriously.

Enjoy yourself! Eliminate anything that does not fulfill your innate sexual desire. Sense it. Sense it. Please do not concern yourself with your appearance or the opinions held by others about you. Effectively permit the innate desire to exert full dominion over your cognizance and physical being.

Enable your physique to communicate to your intellect the words to articulate at this present moment. When expressing your desires, kindly communicate them to him. And subsequently, adopt a calm demeanor and embrace acceptance. Completely surrender to the fervor. You bear the responsibility, my beloved, once you enter this alluring state of mind.

You will remain unaffected by others' opinions as you operate within a distinct domain. He will be keenly cognizant of your desire, with every fiber of his being, particularly those that hold significance. Rely on me. Regardless, he desires this. Your words will elicit a profound response within his mind, reminiscent of a sensual melody replaying persistently. Any aversion he may have had... vanished. I offer my congratulations to you on this significant transition. It is evident that you have embarked upon a new path that promises to be more invigorating and fulfilling, as an alternative to the monotonous and subdued nature of prior sexual experiences.

Got it? Good. In order to have an adequate response when your physical being communicates, please proceed to that location and commence the examination of the aforementioned examples.

Hmm... Are you contemplating the notion, 'Implementing this may prove more challenging than expressing it verbally'? Does it still instill a sense of trepidation within you, the prospect of engaging in provocative dialogue with your partner? That is totally normal. Please continue accompanying me and engage in further discussion to determine if you can acclimate to the concept before fully committing. Rest assured.

Release yourself from fear

Fear serves as a deterrent for the majority of individuals, impeding them from expressing their desired degree of profanity. It is likely that at some juncture, you may have desired to convey explicit instructions regarding your preferences and desires in the realm of intimate encounters. Expressing oneself in a sensual manner provides the opportunity to articulate these specific instructions, enabling effective communication of your desires. You were impeded by a certain factor, yet that hindrance has become redundant. Men have no inclination for the existence of such a barrier. Certainly not! It is imperative that women participate in both the installation and removal of it.

A prevalent occurrence is the inhibition of open expression, which may stem from one's sexual orientation or other influential determinants. It is imperative that you reflect upon the reasons behind your reluctance to express your thoughts and conduct yourself in such a manner.

- Are you of the belief that he will merely find amusement in your situation?

- Do you experience feelings of discomfort related to your sexual orientation?

- May I inquire if your lack of confidence is the sole reason for this?

Individuals will halt their progress before it even commences due to these three principal factors, consequently establishing a foundation for an eventual downfall. Embrace your inner warrior, display courage, and persist in order to explore the intense sensual pleasure that can arise from engaging in explicit communication with your partner.

You may have apprehensions concerning sexual activity. The practice of stigmatizing individuals based on their sexual behavior is pervasive, yet it is crucial to embrace and celebrate one's own sexual expression. We have been designed to derive pleasure from engaging in sexual activity, therefore, it is inherently inherent and in line with our nature. Do not feel ashamed of embracing your sexuality. Instead, assert control over it, and engaging in explicit communication can facilitate this empowerment. Accepting your sexuality in the bedroom will have a transformative impact on your experiences. You must assume responsibility for it as the magnificent deity of sensuality that you embody.

The most effective course of action for individuals experiencing a lack of confidence is to bravely overcome the apprehension hindering their progress. I am unaware of any person engaging in vulgar language during their initial verbal interaction. You develop self-assurance through engaged in risqué conversation. It is logical to assume that individuals refrain from walking until ensuring their ability to complete a 10-mile run, correct? Be a little silly. One must initiate the process and advance accordingly. Misbehaving young lady, I find myself in a similar situation. It appears that you are eager to engage in explicit conversation only once you possess a certain level of self-assurance. Take that decisive step forward, and assume a position of dominance over your opponent.

It shall not have an impact on his viewpoint.

Do you have apprehensions that he might derive amusement and reach the conclusion that you came across as unintelligent? That is highly improbable unless you are in the company of an untruthful individual. In the event that you are, it may be advisable for you to depart promptly. merely a thought.

It is advisable to communicate your preferences, desires, and boundaries to male individuals, articulating your preferences, forms of gratification, desired actions, and mutual reciprocation. Undoubtedly, when it comes to men, the nature of sexual encounters tends to be predominantly unprotected and without any barriers. Do you believe that he desires to embrace you tenderly, delicately caress you, and shower you with sweet, affectionate affection? That book exhibits complete dissimilarity. That particular style of intimate encounters is incongruous with engaging in explicit and provocative verbal communication. When a woman becomes aware that her partner is highly desirous of engaging in sexual intercourse, and she shares the same inclination, she ought to engage in sexually explicit communication. Indeed, there is a distinction to be made, and notwithstanding the facade he may assume, it is highly probable that he aligns with the latter category. He is merely acting in your best interest by carrying out that action. My pleasure.

Please be aware that engaging in explicit conversation will not alter his perception of you. If such an eventuality were to occur, the resulting consequences would be advantageous. He will not unfairly pass judgment upon you for this matter. Should you engage in sexual activity with your partner, it is imperative that you place your trust in him and feel secure in his presence. Regardless of whether or not you express the belief that he should forcefully remove your wet underwear while bending you over a table, his attention and affection towards you will remain unchanged; he will either prioritize you or have strong feelings for you.

One should observe a favorable alteration in their communication upon adopting a deceptive approach. In the event that an individual becomes enthused, it is likely that they will display a smile. That smiling expression is not the subdued laughter that you fear it to be. He is likely envisioning this occasion repeatedly in his mind, and he may be contemplating whether your statement is intended humorously or if you genuinely authorize him to proceed with your request. He contemplates, "Is this event occurring?" as he starts to gaze vacantly. Oh, you are familiar with the saying.

Don your protective armor

Whilst this may appear trivial, donning your armor may imbue you with added assurance when engaging in more explicit discourse. You may be curious as to the nature of your armor. That\\\'s pretty straightforward. All items that elicit a sense of sensuality are encompassed in our offerings. The most effective approach to overcoming the uncomfortable phase of introducing explicit language into one's intimate interactions is to cultivate a sense of allure and self-assurance.

It is remarkable how donning provocative attire can evoke a sense of mischievousness and awaken the rebellious nature within oneself. If necessary, you may choose to let your alter ego assume control. I extend a cordial invitation for them to accompany me. When one is unburdened by the concerns of the tangible realm, it becomes considerably more effortless to direct one's attention towards the immediate moment. This represents your envisioned utopian society. You have the freedom to pursue your desired identity and engage in activities that bring pleasure to your physique.

Irrespective of whether you choose to wear a bra and pant set or opt for complete lingerie, which may include various role playing outfits, it holds no significant bearing. It should solely evoke sensations of warmth, self-assurance, and allure. Your choice of attire should never induce feelings of inadequacy, therefore if you do not prefer it, simply refrain from wearing it. Ensuring that your hair is in optimal condition and that your makeup is carefully applied proves advantageous. Although the act of revealing your full nudity to your partner typically proves effective in arousing them, you may require additional measures to cultivate a sense of assurance and confidence before proceeding. Consequently, it is deemed your protective shield as you combat pheromones, acquire the art of eloquence, and triumph over the boundless peaks of pleasure that undoubtedly await you.

If it is necessary for you to inquire with him

It is advisable to enhance sexual spontaneity with your partner by incorporating explicit communication strategies during intimate moments. However, if such methods make you feel uneasy, a more direct and open approach can involve candidly discussing your partner's thoughts and preferences regarding explicit language within the bedroom. It results in minimal discomfort among male individuals. In general, women tend to encounter feelings of unease in such situations.

The most challenging aspect lies in identifying a suitable opportunity to approach him, hence it is advisable that you simply proceed with the action. If one were to approach the situation gradually by adhering to the subsequent guidelines, they will promptly ascertain his lack of interest. He may narrow his eyes or prohibit your progress (ouch!). Nevertheless, the occurrence of such an event is highly improbable. You can anticipate him to encourage further elaboration from you. Prepare, my beloved.

Please proceed with the task at hand.

Whether you choose to commence directly with instances of explicit conversation, progress through the incremental exercises presented on the subsequent page, or first obtain his explicit consent, the order of approach is inconsequential. The foremost priority lies in initiating intimate and explicit discourse within the confines of the bedroom, which would be beneficial for both parties involved. This activity serves as an excellent means of fostering mutual acquaintance and ensuring ongoing engagement to prevent monotony. Engage in intimate dialogue at the earliest opportunity with the intention of deepening your connection. Inhale deeply, determine your preferred approach, and allow that mischievous side to be unleashed.

Once you have the ability to quieten the inner voice that urges you to embrace and embody your sexuality to the fullest, you will experience an enhanced sense of well-being. By inducing a state of insanity in him, the desired outcome will naturally be achieved within a brief period. Even in the case of engaging in derogatory speech, repetition will lead to mastery, as is the case with all pursuits.

Gaining Insight Into A Woman's Desires

The profound inquiry that has eluded numerous individuals is: 'What is the true desire of a woman?' Women, to a significant extent, present themselves as enigmatic entities, harboring concealed sentiments within the depths of their souls. Many spouses frequently express dissatisfaction with their inadequate comprehension of their partners, even after an extended period of married life. What is the underlying truth behind this enigma that has become a hindrance in a relationship?

There exist assertive and demanding women, as well as wives who frequently nag and assert their authority over their husbands. However, it is important to note that these instances are rare exceptions, often exploited as comedic material to belittle women and stroke the egos of men. This perpetuates the false impression that women are solely responsible for the challenges encountered within relationships. Females, as a whole, tend to demonstrate limited openness when it comes to their emotions, as they are socialized in a manner that prioritizes the needs and concerns of others over their own.

Change is an enduring element in the life of a woman, and following marriage, a woman must acclimate herself to unfamiliar individuals and accustom herself to unfamiliar environments. Frequently, a woman sacrifices various aspects of her life, including her residence, relationship with her parents, personal comfort, established lifestyle, and priorities, to be in the company of her spouse. Men experience a comparative advantage in this matter, as there is minimal disparity in life after marriage. While adapting to an entirely unfamiliar reality in the name of amour, there is minimal space for individual aspirations. In accordance with societal expectations, this is considered the customary standard that each woman is expected to adhere to; however, implementing this can be challenging.

Throughout the courtship process, men spare no effort in courting their beloved, showering them with affection, indulgence, and ample attention. Once married, men often become complacent with their wives and feel the need for special occasions to demonstrate their affection for their partner. As time elapses, gentlemen gradually fail to remember their anniversaries and their wife's birthday. When women become agitated about these matters, men perceive them as being too insignificant to warrant consideration. Females possess an inherent inclination towards emotional responsiveness, wholeheartedly dedicating themselves to retaining intricacies related to personal spheres, including birthdays, anniversaries, or the inaugural encounter.

Women seek sincerity in a gentleman; they frequently harbor concerns regarding a man's demeanor as a result of previous relationships.

Another characteristic that women seek in a man is intellectual prowess. There is a limited number of women who are interested in going out with individuals who lack intelligence. Many individuals aspire to be with a man who would elicit admiration from others. They seek an individual capable of showcasing their academic qualifications, such as college degrees or achievements on the honor roll. The third pivotal element pertains to an individual's financial status. Unless a woman is deeply in love, she is unlikely to be interested in pursuing a romantic relationship with a financially insolvent man.

A woman will exhibit devotion to a man in the event that he encounters a financial crisis subsequent to the establishment of their relationship. However, initially, she would desire the presence of some form of financial stability. Ladies value a certain level of amusement, desiring their partner to elicit laughter from others. Hence, a reserved individual does not fulfill the romantic ideals of all women. They desire for their acquaintances, family members, and loved ones to be filled with amusement and laughter by the individual they support. Another aspect that women seek in a man is his demeanor and courtesy.

No woman desires to engage in a romantic relationship with an individual who, during the initial encounter, explicitly requests her to contribute monetarily. Ladies desire their companions to exhibit courteous behavior and adhere to proper etiquette. It is necessary for them to feel confident they can take their partner out with other friends and not feel embarrassed. Women, too, desire to experience a physical attraction towards a man. Therefore, it could be advantageous for gentlemen to consider the application of a sophisticated fragrance, while, simultaneously, giving careful attention to their attire. The choice of a man's vehicle model is likewise of significance.

Unwavering affection, nurturance, comprehension, reverence, reliance, and integrity encompass a mere slice of a woman's desires, yet there exists a myriad of other facets that contribute to her sense of fulfillment. The enigmatic nature encompassing women is what consistently captivates men. Please consider taking some personal time to reconnect with your fondness for your significant other.

Hinduism's View Of Divine Sex

A considerable number of individuals adhere to the path of Tantra in their pursuit of spiritual connection with the divine. Every aspect of your life has received the blessings of the divine, and this extends to your sexual experiences as well. One will have the opportunity to establish a connection with the divine and transcendental realm solely during the act of engaging in intimate relations with one's partner, as this is the primary means by which one demonstrates reverence and encounters the inherent immortality that resides within the human body. The teachings of Tantra firmly assert that divinity resides within every individual, with a masculine essence in men and a feminine essence in women. This implies that your physical form is the receptacle for immortality. In order to attain the essential levels of intelligence that are available to you, it will be necessary for you to let go of this facade. Your self-assurance will be enhanced when your partner is observing you attentively and you are reciprocating with utmost respect. Once you gain sight of this aspect within yourself, only then will you be afforded the opportunity to perceive the celestial essence that resides equally in others, unequivocally.

At present, we shall embark on the journey of acquiring knowledge and discerning the celestial essence that resides within you. You will have the opportunity to acknowledge the divine presence within your own being and that of your partner as well. This constitutes the epitome of Tantric sexual practices. You will also be able to embark on a path towards increased enlightenment. This section pertains to information regarding diverse deities renowned within the realm of Tantric teachings.

The Designations 'Deity' and 'Divine Being'

As previously mentioned, the teachings of Tantra stipulate that it is imperative to accord utmost reverence and respect to both men and women, perceiving them as divine beings, comparable to deities and goddesses. This is intended to ensure that you not only embody the concept of perpetuity, but also approach your collaboration with the same perspective. Currently, you have the opportunity to appropriately value and esteem your partner. This will also ensure that one can acknowledge the power that resides within the universe.

The deities predominantly venerated in the practice of Tantric sex are perceived as beings brimming with luminosity. They represent distinct forces akin to interpersonal linkages. Alternative terms commonly employed to refer to celestial entities and female deities encompass Deva and Devi, ecclesiastic and priestess, and Daka and Dakini respectively. It is widely acknowledged that these deities possess both power and wisdom. This level of intensity also manifests itself within your physical being. This projection fundamentally hinges upon the divergent ethical principles and distinctive characteristics inherent in your persona.

The term "Goddess" has frequently been employed within the context of Tantra. It is utilized to illustrate a woman who is connected with the feminine energy inherent within her being. The inherent importance of this term generally denoted a woman who was nurturing and resilient. A man is not referred to as God due to the perception of God as a supreme entity in various religions. There exist several religions and some traditions that acknowledge the possibility of individuals attaining divinity or goddesshood through making certain alterations to themselves. Nevertheless, the principles of Tantric sexuality suggest that each individual possesses an inherent celestial essence since birth, which is unalterable.

Tantric sex serves to convey the notion that regardless of one's race, religion, or social status, there exists an inherent divinity within every individual. By employing the metaphor of likening a woman to a deity, one is effectively acknowledging her inherent femininity, encompassing qualities of endearment, grace, allure, and nurturing. Only when a woman embraces her qualities and recognizes her true identity can she earn her own self-respect and gain the respect of those around her. By attending to an individual with reverence, one acknowledges and appreciates their innate qualities as a protector, a source of healing, a provider, and a symbol of strength. It is imperative for him to recognize and appreciate these inherent qualities within himself, as only then will his peers truly hold him in high regard. You may possess familiarity with these attributes, or they may potentially reside within you, awaiting discovery.

Discern Your Roles and Qualities

When embarking on the journey of exploring Tantric sex, it is crucial to first identify the deities or goddesses that personify your being. In order to accomplish this, it is imperative that you acknowledge your fundamental qualities and the multitude of roles you undertake in your existence. Do you consider yourself to possess exceptional abilities? Can I safely assume that you are interested? Would it be accurate to describe you as an entrepreneur? Is it accurate to state that you are truly exceptional? Et cetera. You have the ability to document all of your responses to such inquiries. In order to streamline the process, you have the option of creating a composition or utilizing the technique of mind-mapping. Position an image of oneself at the center of a sheet, then proceed to articulate and elaborate upon the various qualities and traits that one believes oneself possesses.

Once you have collected information regarding the various deities and goddesses provided in the preceding section, you may compile a record of the gods with whom you align yourself. For instance, if you have expressed that you possess innovative qualities, you might draw parallels between yourself and deities such as Shiva or Ares. If one perceives themselves to be charming, they may proceed to document the appellation of Aphrodite.

Redirect Your Focus Beyond the Surface Level

It is highly likely that you are familiar with the famous adage 'never judge hastily.' It is a saying that has undoubtedly permeated public consciousness at some juncture. We generally tend to assign or select an individual primarily based on their physical appearance, attire, or even their occupation. You might have uttered phrases such as 'she is excessively slender' or 'he is excessively brief.' It is likely that you scrutinized an individual's financial situation before consenting to accompany them on a social outing. Regardless, Tantra is concerned with shaping an individual's character rather than focusing on superficial qualities. To fully appreciate the divine essence within your partner, it is essential to adhere to three fundamental principles.

The first step involves recognizing the presence of perpetual existence within oneself. The next step entails comprehending and discerning the divine qualities present within your partner as well. It is essential to strive for a harmonious balance between the masculine and feminine energies inherent in the divine beings. The third phase entails the incorporation of these deities within oneself, accomplished through the bond fostered with one's significant other. This will facilitate the establishment of the essential rapport between the two parties and enable you to attain a higher degree of satisfaction.

What is the importance of displaying admiration towards one another?

Every person experiences an increased sense of happiness upon the realization that they are being acknowledged. It is an extraordinary sensation to be appreciated by those individuals in your immediate vicinity. Are you familiar with the sensation one experiences when they are being observed by another individual? When one endeavors to apprehend you? Tantric sex revolves around the act of revering oneself and one's partner equally. This does not entail that you should mindlessly idolize one another. It essentially denotes the necessity for both individuals to reciprocate unwavering affection towards one another. Complete adoration does not entail exerting authority over one another. It merely suggests the notion of mutually striving to maximize contentment for all parties involved.

Once you embark upon the Tantric sex journey, you will discover the immense pleasure derived from receiving affirming remarks about oneself, and in turn, you will feel compelled to consistently express admiration for your partner. This highlights the significance of holding your partner in high esteem and showing deep respect towards them.

Acquiring Knowledge about the Deities "

Numerous male and female deities, including goddesses, can be observed across a range of civilizations worldwide, such as those in Egypt, Greece, Rome, and India. These celestial entities and deities predominantly originate from a bygone era. Allow us to acquaint ourselves with the diverse pantheon of goddesses.

A significant proportion of the divine goddesses regularly attain the pinnacle of fertility and vitality. Regardless, they are also regarded as bewitching individuals who seduce their companions and engage in sexual acts with them. Currently, we shall uncover information regarding two primary goddesses, through which you may discern certain aspects that resonate with your own being.

Aphrodite:

Aphrodite is regarded as the most revered deity among the pantheon of Greek goddesses. She reaches the pinnacle of excellence, desire, love, and sensuality. She also aspires to companionship. Aphrodite frequently receives communication from avian creatures, floral blossoms, diminutive canines, and even cetaceans. As per Roman mythology, she is referred to as Venus. In the folklore of ancient Rome, she represents the embodiment of virtue.

Artemis:

She is regarded as the deity associated with the pursuit. Artemis is a divinity revered in Ancient Greek mythology, and she ascends to the celestial body known as the moon, embodying purity as a goddess of virginity. She exhibits the qualities of a formidable warrior and skilled tracker, serving as the counterpart to Ares, the divine deity of warfare.

Athena:

The deity of shrewdness and knowledge. She serves as the patron deity of Athens. Athena is commonly associated with the qualities of technique and arrangement.

Juno:

Depending on the Greek or Roman rendition of mythology, Juno or Hera is regarded as a matronly figure characterized by nurturing and tranquil qualities.

Deities of the Hindu Tradition:

In both India and Nepal, a multitude of goddesses exist, each holding immense importance and reverence. Each of these goddesses is accorded reverence and fulfillment of distinct roles. The primordial deities are alluded to in this context.

Durga is revered as the universal mother, encompassing the essence of all manifestations. Tara's character embodies both astuteness and graciousness, which is manifested in her actions and demeanor. Lakshmi assumes the divine embodiment of wealth and prosperity. Saraswati is regarded as the deity presiding over various forms of artistic expression and aptitude. Kali attains a peak of both excellence and intensity. She also serves as the protector of the realm.

Deities from Diverse Cultural Backgrounds

Every religion is comprised of a multitude of celestial entities and deities. These celestial entities often possess a divine counterpart in the form of a goddess. Diverse societies hold reverence for a multitude of deities. They collectively attain immense caliber and strength and are often regarded as extraordinary beings. This segment explores a diverse range of deities from different religious traditions. At this moment, you are given the opportunity to discern and highlight either your own attributes or those of your associate.

Deities of the Hindu Faith:

Lord Shiva, an immensely potent deity, and Lord Vishnu, considered as the embodiment of divine reflection, encompass the pantheon of Hindu gods. There exist diverse manifestations of Lord Shiva, accompanied by numerous depictions of his enigmatic aspects. Shakti is in companionship with Lord Shiva. The union of Master Shiva and

Shakti produces an innovative union that culminates in the manifestation of pure energy. Ganesh holds significance as a renowned deity; he embodies the representation of a youthful being adorned with the majestic head of an elephant. Master Ganesh is renowned for removing obstacles and promoting contentment. Master Rama and Sita are regarded as a highly revered couple across India, embodying an ideal partnership that epitomizes the harmony that ought to prevail between a husband and wife.

Greek deities:

There exist numerous deities in Greek mythology, acclaimed for their exceptional strength and prowess, leading to their widespread renown. Zeus is widely regarded as the supreme being, holding the title of the sovereign ruler over all domains and epitomizing extraordinary dominance as the quintessential alpha figure. Eros is commonly referred to as Cupid, assuming the form of a cherubic young man, whose nature is often mischievous as he incessantly imparts the arrows of affection upon those in his proximity. He is the divine being associated with the attribute of love. Dionysus represents the deity of desire in both Greek and Roman mythology. In accordance with the narratives, he consistently pursued the company of women and relished consuming a copious amount of wine. Indeed, he undoubtedly embodies the supreme essence of passion.

CHAPTER FOUR

EARLY CHILDHOOD(2-5 years)

You are now required to communicate to them the appropriate nomenclature of the physical components and their respective functions.

Females commonly possess a vulva, whereas males typically possess buttocks, nasal appendages, appendages for manipulating objects, and so forth. Males and females exhibit inherent differences, while still sharing commonalities.

It is socially acceptable to embrace diversity and acknowledge the inherent variation in our physical appearances. Given the extensive range of emotions we possess and our ability to perceive them physically, it can be inferred that our bodies possess the capacity to convey our psychological experiences to us.

Privacy

Specific parts of the body are considered private, and should not be exposed to the general public.

The concept of distinct private and public locations and time periods can be challenging for young individuals to comprehend due to its variability. For instance, it may be considered acceptable for your child to be unclothed in the privacy of your home when their grandmother is present; however, it would be deemed inappropriate when there is a plumber present.

To uphold the privacy of others. For instance, in the event that the lavatory door is shut, individuals should politely knock and seek permission to enter.

They have a right to privacy as well, such as during moments of attending to personal needs like using the restroom, bathing, or dressing.

This pertains to the concept of reserving discussions on human bodies for intimate settings such as one's residence or in the presence of their guardians, as opposed to engaging in such conversations in public spaces such as playgrounds or schoolyards.

It is deemed appropriate to engage in physical contact with one's genitalia, but it is important to exercise discretion and adhere to proper circumstances.

Establish limitations pertaining to sexual activity involving the genitals. Elucidate the fact that the act of touching one's genitals can generate pleasurable sensations, however, it is considered a private behavior akin to toileting, and should only be pursued in a secluded environment, such as a bedroom.

If your child engages in touching their genital area during social situations, it is advised to respectfully remind them to refrain from placing their hands inside their trousers. Please refrain from exaggerating the significance of their actions, as they engage in them to cultivate a sense of security. In due course, they will surpass it!

Observed engaging in a game of 'doctor' with a peer (exchanging glances at intimate body parts), exhaling audibly, tactfully intervening, urging them to dress, and redirecting their attention towards a different plaything or pastime. Subsequently, matters pertaining to privacy and limitations concerning physical contact may be discussed.

All organisms engage in reproduction, whereby plants disperse seeds, canines give birth to offspring, and humans procreate. Gradually begin identifying instances of reproduction as you observe them.

A child undergoes development within the woman's womb, also known as the uterus or the gestational sac, and eventually the specifics of this process will be elaborated upon. Both a male and a female are necessary in order to procreate.

The process of human reproduction involves the merger of genetic material from a male, in the form of sperm cells, and a female, in the form of egg cells, resulting in the creation of offspring. Often, the inquiry of one's origin is the initial query posed by young individuals.

The process by which an embryo matures and grows within the womb of a female human. Maintain utmost simplicity— their sole desire pertains to core principles. The details are presented at a substantially later stage.

If children wish to acquire knowledge regarding the process of childbirth, one can provide a concise explanation that states that the baby is delivered either through the woman's abdominal region or through her vaginal canal.

The act of procreation is reserved for adults and not intended for individuals of youthful age. Make it a habit to consistently remind them of this fact during each discussion.

Ownership of the human body and tactile engagement

They possess sovereignty over their own physical being and possess the prerogative to establish boundaries concerning physical contact, which includes yourself.

It is considered inappropriate to initiate physical contact or embrace another person without their consent, and the same applies reciprocally.

On occasion, there may be justifiable circumstances for an adult to examine or make contact with their own physique, as would be the case with a medical professional. We do not engage in the harboring of undisclosed information pertaining to our physical selves. Confidential information may pertain to unexpected occurrences and presents.

They have the ability to communicate with you about any matter that elicits negative or positive emotions.

The assistance they necessitate

Preschool-age children represent the most uncomplicated age group when it comes to education. They possess an insatiable thirst for knowledge, akin to empty sponges yearning to absorb information about myriad subjects. If a rational explanation eludes them, individuals are inclined to employ their imagination to construct a justification.

Prepare yourself for the likelihood of having to repeat instructions, as children are prone to forgetting and may not fully grasp or only partially hear what you initially communicate to them. Do not overlook the importance of inquiring about their intended meaning in order to provide an apt response.

You aim to establish yourself as their primary reservoir of expertise. This encompasses the virtue of honesty and attending to their inquiries regarding infants.

Responding to your child conveys the notion that they can openly communicate with you about any subject matter, instilling the belief that you are a trustworthy and reliable source of information.

This is a favorable development, especially as they commence engaging with their peers.

If you find it challenging to find the appropriate language, there are numerous exceptional resources in the form of sex education books that you can make use of. They disseminate the information and are composed in a manner suitable for the intended age group. Furthermore, at this stage of development, children fail to perceive the presence of an educational tome within the assortment of literature you skim through prior to sleep each evening.

Chapter Four

Commencing a dialogue amidst existing social unease

Comment on an Individual Matter

It shall be apparent to you that every individual you encounter possesses a distinctive element about them; be it an embellishment, a peculiar attire, or even a tattoo. These narratives recount a story pertaining to a single individual.

Whenever you take notice of and commend them, it serves as an impetus for initiating a conversation. For instance, you may initiate a discussion by expressing:

I must say, that pendant is truly exquisite. What type of stone is it?

Nice shirt! Are you a fan of the Grateful Dead?

Please refrain from commenting on intimate aspects of one's appearance, such as asking, "Is that your natural hair color?" or remarking, "You must work out extensively!"

Once you have elicited a response, make certain that you have an additional statement prepared. This will provide you with a conventional platform to initiate a dialogue and, subsequently, foster a connection with the individual you have just encountered, even if the connection only lasts for a brief period.

Present an ensuing narrative that reveals a glimpse of personal information pertaining to yourself. As an example, once the person addresses your initial question, you may revisit the topic by stating something along the lines of: "

I observed a similar pendant at a jewelry establishment last week.

My father was a truly devoted fan of the Grateful Dead. During my childhood, he dedicated an increased amount of time to visit them.

\\\"I love tattoos. I have been contemplating the idea of acquiring one; however, I am uncertain about the particular option to choose. "Why did you make a decision to choose Yoda as your final choice?

These claims will aid in establishing a connection with the individual and maintaining the flow of conversation. I kindly request that you bear in mind that the goal is not to articulate the perfect statement or adhere rigidly to a particular approach, but rather to sustain the ongoing dialogue.

Systematic guidelines for inquiring about follow-up topics in casual conversations

Kindly inquire if we have previously had the opportunity to meet.

This exceptional ice breaker has the potential to be effective under optimal circumstances. If one were to express, "You emanate an undeniable sense of authenticity. Have we, by any chance, crossed paths before?" it facilitates the acquisition of information regarding the individual, thus enabling the progression of the conversation.

For example, in the event that you inquire someone about their secondary school and discover that you both attended a comparable institution, you may proceed by presenting a fact such as, "I participated in the marching band."

"Have you engaged in playing a musical instrument?" Assuming you inquire about someone's occupation and acknowledge having witnessed them in that particular context, it presents an opportunity for you to establish a connection by expressing appreciation, such as "I greatly admire that particular Starbucks establishment!" While the other individual shares personal information with you, it is permissible to embark on intriguing tangents. Please bear in mind that the intention is not simply to ascertain if you have encountered one another before, but rather to establish a genuine understanding of the other person.

Injecting humor to create a more relaxed atmosphere

Another remarkable approach to initiate a conversation with individuals in your vicinity is to make an observation about the shared surroundings. A touch of levity can be remarkably effective in this context. As an example, let's say you find yourself in an auditorium and you happen to observe that your teacher bears a striking resemblance to the character Harry Potter. In this situation, you may choose to privately convey to the person next to you, "Doesn't he bear a resemblance to Harry Potter?"

Maintain a positive editorial tone at all times, avoiding any expressions of timidity or criticism. You hold the belief that the other individual ought to be inclined towards participating in the humor along with you. Perhaps you could revisit your previous comment concerning your teacher by stating, "I ponder the whereabouts of Hedwig."

Humor can be precarious when interacting with individuals with whom one has limited familiarity, thus employing this approach to initiate a conversation can be precarious. However, if you do happen to encounter someone who genuinely appreciates your sense of humor, it can mark the beginning of a wonderful friendship. If one individual does not yield a positive response, the approach may prove effective with another person. The greater amount of practice you engage in, the easier it will become to communicate with an unfamiliar individual. Over time, you will become increasingly confident and won't need to rely on tricks to initiate a conversation and ensure its success.

Have a significant impact on the Discussion

One might become disengaged from the discussion due to a combination of excessive anxiety and lack of conversational experience. However, a recent report has revealed that individuals suffering from social anxiety exhibit a diminished inclination to actively engage in discussions. Consequently, they are less favored in comparison to their counterparts. Therefore, it is imperative to uphold your end of a dialogue once initiated. Plenty of individuals are comfortable engaging in this activity with acquaintances, but they exhibit reluctance when it comes to involving unfamiliar individuals. Their prevailing apprehension hinders their self-realization and hampers the expression of their true nature.

Overcome challenges in engaging in discussions

Lacking in specific interpersonal skills can hinder your ability to engage in meaningful conversations, particularly if it gives the impression of hostility. For example, studies indicate that individuals experiencing social apprehension tend to frequently maintain eye contact during conversations. Enhancing your ability to visually engage while conversing can help portray a sense of openness and amiability. This will enhance the likelihood of individuals responding to your efforts to initiate a conversation. If you believe that you lack the requisite communication skills and experience to be a proficient conversationalist, self-improvement manuals and professional guidance can aid you in developing them.

Extra: Typical Circumstances Involving Intimacy (and Strategies for Approaching Them Candidly)

At a certain juncture within your sexual experiences, it is inevitable that you will encounter one or more of the subsequent situations:

Sexual dysfunction

Sexual dysfunction encompasses challenges related to sexual response, arousal, orgasm, desire, or discomfort. It may arise from diverse factors such as heightened stress levels, consumption of tobacco or alcohol, the use of specific medications, underlying physiological conditions, or challenges within interpersonal relationships.

Discussing sexual dysfunction is crucial as failing to do so may lead your partner to mistakenly believe they are at fault, potentially causing harm to your relationship.

If your partner is encountering sexual difficulties, it is advisable that you:

Kindly request an opportunity for a calm and affectionate conversation with your partner, ensuring to select an appropriate setting and timing.

Refrain from assigning fault to either your partner or yourself for the current circumstances in the bedroom. Inquire with your partner regarding their emotional state and inquire if there are any actions they would appreciate your assistance with. Please ensure to explicitly acknowledge that we are unified in this endeavor.

It is advisable to refrain from utilizing the term "performance" in discussions related to sexual activity. Utilizing this term can create a sense of undue pressure on your counterpart to achieve specific objectives. Refer to it by its accurate terminology: "engage in sexual intercourse."

Once you and your partner have reached a stage where you can engage in a candid and forthright dialogue, propose the idea of scheduling a medical consultation to gain a better comprehension of the situation.

In the event that you are the individual experiencing the dysfunction within the partnership, it would be advisable to engage in an open and honest conversation with your significant other, effectively articulating the impact of the sexual issue on your well-being. Offer reassurance to your partner that, despite the prevailing issue, your sentiments of yearning towards them remain unwavering, and that you possess the capability to express this affection through alternate means. For example, if you are experiencing difficulties attaining an erection, oral stimulation provided to your partner may be considered.

When facing a period of stagnation

A romantic or intimate stagnation may arise when one becomes entrenched in a state of complacency, adhering to the belief that there is no need for change in their sexual experiences.

One may have experimented with a particular approach, found it appealing, and subsequently persisted with it. It can be quite common to become trapped in repetitive sexual routines, particularly if there has been a lack of discussion regarding individual preferences from the initial stages.

This situation has the potential to engender tedium and a diminished sense of sexual fervor due to the predictable nature of each occurrence.

If you find yourself in a cycle of stagnation:

Kindly engage with your partner at an opportune moment and in a suitable setting.

Don't assign any blame. Express to your partner that while you genuinely appreciate engaging in sexual activity together, you believe that introducing some variety has the potential to enhance the pleasure and satisfaction derived from it.

When you are confident that your partner is attentive, propose engaging in activities to enhance and invigorate the relationship. One may avail themselves of online resources or peruse printed publications to discover activities that both parties might be inclined to explore. Please ensure that you inquire with your partner if there are any preferences or desires they would like to explore as well.

In certain instances, particularly if you have pursued various attempts but continue to find yourself trapped in a repetitive pattern, it may be advisable to seek consultation from a qualified professional in the field of sexual therapy.

When one is not experiencing the desired inclination

As enjoyable as the act of sexual intercourse may be, candidly speaking, it can also be physically demanding, and occasions arise when one may lack the necessary vitality to fully engage in such activities. There is no issue with this.

Should one of you be prepared while the other remains unprepared, the sexual encounter shall prove physically dissatisfying and devoid of any emotional bond. Engaging in such sexual encounters may lead to the development of emotional detachment, a regrettable outcome as a mere expression of disinterest could have sufficed in such situations.

Prior communication with your partner is essential in this regard. Do refrain from permitting the escalation of intimate activities with your partner before conveying your disinterest in engaging. If, upon returning home, you find yourself genuinely unable to engage in sexual activity, openly communicate to your partner that you have experienced a prolonged and exhausting day, and your current inclination is solely towards seeking rest. A compassionate companion will comprehend, as both men and women encounter such situations to an equivalent extent.

It is advised to maintain a direct and honest approach in order to reassure your partner that they are not the cause of the issue. Please arrange a new meeting time in a professional manner, and ensure that the revised schedule is strictly adhered to.

One could express it in a formal tone as follows: "An alternative phrasing could be, 'I have deep affection for you and desire physical intimacy, yet my beloved, today has been quite challenging.'" I am in need of some rest urgently, as soon as possible. Let's reschedule for tomorrow. Rest assured, you will highly appreciate what awaits you in the future."

What is the desired frequency?

It is not uncommon to become disoriented amidst one's hectic routines, leading to a moment of realization that a considerable amount of time has transpired since engaging in sexual activities. In the event of this occurrence, promptly prioritize carving out time for open communication, lest your intimate relationship becomes overshadowed by the demands and obligations of daily life.

Initiate the dialogue by expressing to your partner your perception that the frequency of your intimate encounters has been insufficient recently, and convey your desire to establish a specific weekly frequency for engaging in sexual activity. Inquire of your partner regarding their perspectives and emotions pertaining to that matter.

Deliberating upon the frequency of intimate encounters per week may seem conventional, but occasionally, organizing a timetable for sexual activity can prove to be the solution that revitalizes your relationship.

Discuss the preferable timing for engaging in sexual activity: morning versus evening. You may discover that one individual has a preference for mornings while the other tends to be more inclined towards evenings. Seek a mutual agreement and identify viable solutions as collaborative partners.

One could also consider strategies for adding excitement or innovation. As an illustration, on specific occasions, your significant other may arrange unexpected evenings filled with romance, while you devise activities of a more intimate nature to enhance the experience.

Enriching Your Lexicon Of Indecent Terminology

One of the predominant challenges associated with engaging in explicit conversations is the inclination to become redundant in one's speech. If one discovers that they are consistently reiterating the same term, it may be necessary to consider broadening one's lexicon. Although there are complete phrases later in the book, you have the flexibility to vary them by substituting words according to your preference.

As an illustration, if the expression is "I want your dick inside me," one can readily substitute it with "I desire your prick/rod/cock inside me."

Aroused: Elicited sexual stimulation, experiencing heightened desire, feeling passionate and stimulated, roused with sexual anticipation, thoroughly aroused, experiencing heightened sensuality, being in a state of increased sexual excitement.

Anus: rectum, posterior opening, anal passage, posterior orifice, anal cavity, anal sphincter, anal orifice, anal aperture, anal opening, rectal opening

Mammary glands: bosom, female chest, frontal protuberances, mammary tissue, female bust, feminine curves, feminine bosom, female anatomy, female physique, feminine attributes, female assets, female proportions, female chest area, female mammary region

The clitoris is referred to by various terms such as bean, button, clit, devil's doorbell, fun button, happy button, hooded lady, kernel, love bud, love button, man in the boat, nub, and sweet spot.

Ejaculate: expel seminal fluid, achieve orgasm, release semen, reach climax, discharge, orgasmic release, seminal emission, ejaculatory response, reach sexual climax.

Erection: tumescence, phallus enlargement, achievement of rigidity, engorgement, penile stiffening, manifestation of virility, creation of an elevated state

Engage in sexual activity: engage in intercourse, be intimate, engage in sexual relations, copulate, procreate, engage in sexual congress, engage in sexual intercourse, engage in coitus, consummate a relationship, engage in sexual interaction, engage in sexual contact, engage in a physical connection, engage in a sexual encounter, engage in sexual congress, engage in sexual relations, form a sexual union, engage in sexual acts, engage in a sexual liaison

Engage in self-pleasure: self-stimulate, indulge in solo sexual activity, fondle oneself, engage in personal sexual gratification, manually stimulate one's own genitals, engage in autoeroticism, practice self-gratification, engage in solitary sexual pleasure, partake in self-pleasuring activities, satisfy one's sexual desires in private.

Fellatio: felching, fellating, giving/receiving oral pleasure, performing oral sex, performing fellatio, receiving a blowjob, engaging in oral stimulation, ingesting seminal fluid, orally servicing, administering oral gratification, participating in oral intercourse, indulging in oral activities, performing a phallic act, swallowing ejaculate

Performing cunnilingus, engaging in oral stimulation of the female genitals, providing oral pleasure, bestowing oral gratification, indulging in reciprocal oral intimacy, savoring the taste of a peach, engaging in oral-genital contact, partaking in a delicate meal between the thighs, exploring the art of oral satisfaction, experiencing the delights of oral pleasuring.

Phallus: progenitor, reproductive organ, organ of copulation, amorous shaft, male genitalia, masculine appendage, the unitary optic monster, phallic symbol, vertical structure, male member, male organ, reproductive rod, virile limb, masculine serpent, male genital organ

Semen: seminal fluid, reproductive fluid, ejaculate, sperm, reproductive material, seminal discharge, seminal secretion, male reproductive fluid, male gamete, male reproductive cells, procreative fluid, prostatic fluid, reproductive essence.

Testicles: testes, scrotum, male reproductive organs, genitalia, gonads, male gonads, testicular glands, male reproductive glands, male genitalia, reproductive testes, testicular sac

"Vagina: genital aperture, female reproductive organ, female genitalia, female intimate anatomy, female love tunnel, female reproductive passage, female pleasure center, feminine anatomical structure

Certain words in this collection might appear trivial or absurd to you; however, it is of no consequence. Choose the ones that resonate with you and suit your preferences, and then proceed to incorporate them into your vocabulary.

Initiating Conversations on Erotic Language

Engaging in explicit or sexually suggestive conversation may appear to be... .. Indeed, due to its unclean condition, it may require some additional effort to initiate its operation. If you aspire to possess the eloquence in employing profane language during moments of heightened sensuality, this book shall serve as a valuable resource. However, it is imperative that you first cultivate the necessary confidence to embark on this endeavor.

Do you experience a loss of cognitive function during the performance? Subsequently, here is something to ponder... Endeavor to provide a thorough account of your activities or the actions being performed upon you.

For instance, one may express affection by stating, "I thoroughly enjoy engaging in intimate activities with you." Alternatively, one could describe the pleasurable sensation experienced when engaging in oral stimulation. Elaborate by articulating the specific aspects and sensations that are appreciated during the act. This presents a convenient and accessible approach to commence.

Not all individuals may be at ease with more risqué language, and that is acceptable. Begin with the aspects that naturally align with your abilities, and gradually incorporate a selection of unfamiliar vocabulary at regular intervals. In due course, those expressions will become ingrained within you, leading you to possess proficient skills in engaging in risqué conversation.

Enticement: The Craft of Verbal Communication in Pre-Intimate Interactions

Were you aware that engaging in explicit conversations can commence well before engaging in sexual activities? Engaging in digital communication through texting and phone conversations, or even expressing affectionate remarks to your significant other in the morning, can evoke a heightened sense of excitement and passion.

The act of eagerly anticipating an event or experience holds tremendous power and serves as the ultimate precursor to pleasure. When you inform your significant other about the existence of something extraordinary that awaits them upon their arrival at home tonight, they shall contemplate it throughout the entire day. It is essential to communicate your thoughts to them sufficiently early in the day so as to ignite their passion well in advance of their arrival at home.

A suitable approach would be to express admiration for your partner's attractiveness before they embark on their daily activities. Additionally, it is viable to convey your thoughts to them via text, informing them of your thoughtful considerations. Alternatively, you can communicate a forthcoming itinerary of activities that you intend to engage in together at a later time. Please ensure that you transmit such information via a private message, as opposed to a work email or any other communication medium susceptible to being accessed by others.

Please provide a detailed account of your intended actions towards their person, express your current state of heightened arousal, and convey your impatience in engaging in sexual intercourse. Alternatively, adopt a more nuanced approach and express to your significant other that you engage in self-stimulation while contemplating their presence, expressing uncertainty in your ability to withstand such desires until your next encounter.

Engaging in prelude activities does not necessarily entail physical contact alone. It can also be highly intellectual, and utilizing provocative communication is the ideal means to achieve it.

Engaging in Hands-on Work or Experiencing Gritty Situations

Once an individual is situated in bed, they may find it increasingly feasible to engage in provocative and explicit conversations. You will notice that enhanced levels of arousal in both parties tend to facilitate the effortless expression of words. The subsequent suggestions will assist you in communicating with proficiency.

Be Confident

Uttering meekly that you desire to engage in explicit intimacy with someone until complete oblivion is not an effective approach; therefore, it is advisable to enter this situation with utmost confidence. You possess an inherent allure, and your partner, too, exudes a captivating presence. Hence, this moment presents an ideal opportunity to showcase and celebrate these qualities.

It is generally advisable to initiate conversations by offering gentle praises and gradually progress towards addressing any negative aspects, especially when interacting with someone new. You are uncertain of their potential response, and it has the potential to overwhelm them. This holds especially true in the context of men engaging in explicit communication with women. It may be perceived as inappropriate and unsettling if you immediately use derogatory terms like "bitch," "whore," or "slut" to refer to her.

Watch Your Lover

Does your partner engage in explicit language during intimate conversations? The majority of individuals possess certain inclinations, albeit in varying degrees, and one must closely observe their behavior in order to ascertain their specific sources of arousal. It is possible that they may respond by engaging in explicit conversation, which can be viewed as a strong indication of their enjoyment. Nevertheless, although verbal communication may be absent, nonverbal cues convey substantial meaning. Indicators that your romantic partner derives pleasure from explicit verbal exchanges comprise:

- Accelerated respiration

- Emitting distressful sounds

- Engaging in a slight back curvature - Performing an arching motion with the back - Executing a subtle curvature of the back - Adopting a gentle arch in the back

Engaging in self-stimulation

- Astonishment - Exclamations of surprise - Breathless reactions

- Increased pace of sexual activity.

Non-verbal cues are highly informative, therefore, once acquainted with your partner's preferences, you can increase the amount of actions that align with those preferences. In the event that they do not respond positively, it might be necessary to transition to a more subdued approach.

Fantasize with Them

This opportune moment is ideal for expressing your imaginative desires and formulating innovative plans to pleasure your partner. You may discover that your shared interests extend to similar fantasies. Feel free to engage in open and intimate discussions, wherein you can transform your ideas into stimulating and exhilarating experiences.

One might also consider taking the subsequent measure and actively manifesting their fantasies; nevertheless, that particular subject matter shall be reserved for another literary work. At present, engage in a conversation and deliberate upon potential scenarios where you can express your intentions towards your partner. For instance, if you were in a bustling nightclub where your intimate interaction would go unnoticed, how would you engage in physical contact with the other individual?

Begin gradually and progress systematically" "Initiate the process with caution and gradually enhance" "Commence at a leisurely pace and steadily develop

Effective erotic communication does not immediately progress towards the most explicit language without building up to it. Commence at a moderate pace by expressing phrases such as, "I have a strong desire for you in this moment." Gradually progress towards more intense alternatives. It is imperative for you to possess precise knowledge regarding the specific thoughts and sentiments that elicit a favorable response from your partner. It is possible that you may not be able to progress to the explicit language mentioned later in this book due to your partner's lack of interest.

With that being considered, as your level of arousal intensifies and you become more engrossed in the act at hand, you will discover that verbalizing explicit content becomes increasingly effortless, as your cognitive faculties allocate greater attention to the present activity. The phenomenon of heightened physiological and cognitive response has the potential to elicit remarkable effects within the realm of the human brain. Your partner is apt to be aroused by stimuli that they would typically disregard in a non-aroused state.

Use the Force

The more sexually stimulated both individuals are, the more effortless it will be to engage in explicit conversation and actively listen to explicit language. Upon careful consideration, it is likely that individuals have engaged in certain behaviors impulsively during moments of heightened arousal, which they would not typically engage in under normal circumstances. The aforementioned statement can also be applied to the exchange of explicit language. Therefore, when you become engrossed in intimacy and thoroughly aroused, it is an opportune moment to engage in verbal provocations and demonstrate to your partner the extent of your abilities.

Moreover, the likelihood of encountering rejection or ridicule during sexual intercourse is minimized, as both partners are mutually engaged and the intensity of the intimate experience is heightened. Indeed, you may receive a reciprocal exchange of lewd conversation.

Practice Makes Perfect

Similar to any worthwhile endeavor, engaging in intimate verbal communication necessitates a significant amount of training and persistence. Engage in explicit and suggestive communication with your romantic partner whenever suitable opportunities arise. Engage in it intimately during sexual encounters, remotely through telephone conversations, and in written exchanges through text messages. The greater your efforts, the more proficient you will become.

If one happens to be exceptionally reserved, there is an option to refine one's skills through solitary practice. This approach is most effective when you are deriving satisfaction while speaking, but you may also opt to rehearse in front of a reflective surface. Regardless, the expressions should begin to effortlessly roll off your tongue.

Select Your Preferred Monikers for Pets

It can be quite uncomfortable to abruptly introduce endearments such as "Oh god, baby, yes," particularly if one has not previously referred to their partner using such terms. For certain individuals, devising suitable terms of endearment for their partners can be regarded as a pivotal aspect of readiness in engaging in intimate communication.

It may be advisable to adhere to more traditional terms of endearment, such as baby, honey, lover, and so forth. Alternatively, one could explore more advanced levels of intimacy by referring to their partner as "daddy," "love slave," "master," "mistress," and other similar terms. If you have a deep inclination to adopt vulgar and disrespectful language, terms such as "bitch," "whore," "cum slut," "bastard," and comparable epithets possess the capability to be utilized. It is important to bear in mind that not all individuals appreciate being referred to as a slut, hence it is advisable to assess your audience before using this term extensively.

Intercourse is highly pleasurable and can be a source of great enjoyment, however, engaging in explicit communication significantly enhances the overall experience. Not all individuals will endeavor to engage in explicit language, however, they are truly depriving themselves of a truly remarkable experience. Please proceed with experimenting and determining your own preferences and those of your partner. You might be surprised.

Guidelines For Facilitating A Smooth And Productive Conversation

Do not apprehend the day that you must engage in the conversation with your daughter. On the contrary, anticipate it with enthusiasm, welcome it, and diligently make arrangements for that day. Providing comprehensive sexual education to your child is undoubtedly one of your paramount responsibilities as a parent. You are equipping your daughter for the transition into adolescence and, eventually, maturity. Presented herein are indispensable recommendations that can benefit all parents as they assume this significant duty.

First Tip: Maintain Open Channels of Communication.

It is imperative for your child to have an open line of communication with you wherein she feels comfortable discussing any matter. Establish a conducive setting wherein she will be free from any feelings of fear or embarrassment when seeking clarifications. Always allocate sufficient time to engage in conversations with her, inquire about her daily experiences, and provide her with a safe space to share her personal thoughts. At this developmental phase, adolescent females may express a desire to discuss their emotions regarding males, in addition to the physiological transformations occurring within their bodies. Please ensure that you are prepared for the moment when she chooses to confide in you regarding her infatuation. Please refrain from becoming excessively alarmed and delivering a sermon concerning her perceived youth and ability to experience romantic attachments. Alternatively, it is advisable to foster and promote her engagement in communication, exhibit empathy, extend assistance, and above all, provide suitable guidance.

Guideline #2: Furnish truthful responses

Ensure that you consistently provide your daughter with truthful responses whenever she seeks your guidance on matters related to puberty and sexuality. The individual's decision to approach you demonstrates a profound level of trust, as well as confidence in your ability to provide insight. Do not evade her inquiry or, more significantly, provide a fraudulent response. In order to enhance your ability to address her inquiries more effectively, it is imperative to elucidate the precise nature of her queries. Based on this essential elucidation, proceed to provide her with the requisite response. Furthermore, address each of her inquiries individually. This will facilitate the provision of accurate responses and enhance her capacity to assimilate the new information more efficiently. Furthermore, it is essential to permit her to articulate her inquiries. Allow her an opportunity to express herself. Please refrain from inquiring on her behalf and avoid hasty assumptions. By following these three steps, you will provide your daughter with the answer she requires.

Recommendation #3: Update Your Expertise

One would not engage in armed conflict without the necessary weaponry, would they? Engaging in a discussion about sexuality with your daughter may not be deemed equivalent to engaging in armed conflict, yet it would be highly beneficial for you to be adequately prepared and well-informed for such an important conversation. It is strongly advised that you acquaint yourself with the knowledge of biology, anatomy, and physiology. If you possess a clear understanding of terminology, bodily functions, and processes, you will be capable of furnishing your child with responses that are more precise and unequivocal in nature.

Recommendation #4: Ensure Practicality

When engaging in discussions about reproductive health with your child, ensure that the conversation does not transform into a supplementary lecture on the subject matter. You do not serve as her educator; rather, you fulfill the role of her legal guardian. Engage in a conversation with her pertaining to topics such as menstruation, puberty, and sexual education in a more intimate and tailored manner. Make an effort to refrain from delivering information to her in a manner resembling a scholarly discourse on scientific subjects. Provide pertinent information that she can integrate into her routine, including strategies such as storing supplementary menstrual products in her belongings or school compartment, addressing the matter of accidental stains on her attire while attending school, and effectively managing menstrual discomfort such as cramps.

Recommendation #5: Cease, Engage in Conversation, and Actively Hear

Please ensure to consistently facilitate open lines of communication in both directions. Engage in verbal communication and demonstrate active listening skills. Refrain from solely delivering a monologue and abruptly instructing her to depart. This conversation holds significant importance, therefore it is essential that you establish a connection with your daughter. Provide her with the reassurance that you will consistently be available to lend a listening ear, and that she can seek your counsel whenever necessary.

Guideline #6: Select the Suitable Time and Location

The optimal timeframe for initiating a conversation with your daughter regarding menstruation is typically when she approaches the age range of 8 to 9 years. If you delay any further, she may experience her initial menstrual cycle without being aware of it, which might cause considerable distress. Remember Carrie. When broaching the subject of her initial menstruation, adolescence, and sexuality, it is crucial to ensure she is seated for the conversation. Avoid discussing menstruation with her in public, such as while walking on the street, shopping, or, even worse, during a family gathering. Instead, establish a planned time for this conversation or carefully choose an appropriate moment to address the topic. It is important to ensure that she is comfortably seated, allowing her to fully comprehend the information you will provide.

Ensure that her siblings are not in close proximity, attentively eavesdropping, and prepared to ridicule her. It would be ill-advised to engage in such conversation in the presence of her acquaintances, relatives, and loved ones. Your daughter regards her bedroom as a sanctuary and it would be most suitable to have the conversation in this setting where she will experience the utmost ease and reassurance. Furthermore, one has the ability to mitigate disturbances and diversions.

There are instances of profound connection between a parent and their child. Now would be an opportune moment to engage in a conversation with your daughter regarding her initial menstrual cycle.

Lastly, provide reassurance to your daughter by imparting the understanding that the process of puberty is a universal experience for both genders, and that she is not alone in encountering the physical transformations and intense emotional fluctuations. You may opt to inform her that the process of puberty can be likened to the transformative stage experienced by every butterfly, commonly known as the caterpillar phase. This transitional phase in her life shall come to an end, and she, in due course, shall blossom into a graceful and self-assured woman.

Introducing Fantasies

Both of these phenomena present contrasting characteristics; however, they are perceived through distinct lenses. If one were to inquire about the fantasies harbored by acquaintances, it is likely that the discourse would predominantly center on those fantasies that exist solely in the realm of imagination, as opposed to plausible aspirations. Discussions pertaining to engaging in sexual activities with multiple women simultaneously are often held among men, while acknowledging that although it might be a course of action some individuals are open to exploring, it is less commonly favored by the majority of women. Women are often drawn to the allure of exclusivity and tend to have a preference for safeguarding their possessions without engaging in any form of sharing. Conversely, women frequently exhibit reticence when it comes to divulging their fantasies. If you assemble a gathering of women at a social event that offers products related to sexual pleasure, anticipate a greater likelihood of openness and honesty among them. So, why is it that women are unable to openly acknowledge their genuine emotions to their male counterparts?

It is an undeniable reality that societal norms dictate distinct roles for females and males. Women are held to societal expectations of exhibiting femininity, displaying a refined demeanor, and adhering to a general consensus that discussions surrounding sexuality should be avoided, with an overall belief that actions hold greater significance than mere words. If individuals were approached individually and informed that they were being surveyed regarding their perspectives on sex, it is likely that they would provide more truthful responses. Hence, why do women hesitate to divulge their thoughts to their partners? It is evident that males often have a curiosity to ascertain the origin of this sexual substance. In the event that a woman exudes strong sexual allure, a man may feel inclined to inquire about the number of past partners she has had, and if he measures up to their experiences, as well as whether her behavior has remained consistent across her previous relationships and into the present. It is an exercise in self-aggrandizement, and individuals of male gender struggle to cope with any form of comparative assessment. Women possess a heightened sense of awareness towards the desires of their male partners, even beyond their own comprehension. Recognizing the societal expectation for women to exhibit a certain level of modesty, it is improbable for them to engage in explicit language within intimate settings.

Another intriguing aspect lies in the disparity between women's beliefs concerning the factors that arouse their male partners and men's perceptions of their own arousal triggers. What women and men see as sexy is very different indeed. Hence, you are additionally confronted with the predicament of conforming to your partner's expectations, while simultaneously being subjected to societal norms dictating how women should comport themselves. Nevertheless, if one were to consider the sheer volume of copies of

50 Shades of Grey in circulation, it becomes evident that women possess a latent inclination towards a yearning for adventure, albeit in manners they might hesitate to openly acknowledge.

Why we have fantasies

What is the underlying reason behind our fondness for chocolate? It's the pleasure factor. The veracity of the pleasure, be it genuine or merely a figment of the mind, holds relatively little significance. If you are capable of engaging in open communication with your partner, thereby encouraging them to unveil their secret desires, you might discover mutual surprises that increase your level of comfort towards incorporating provocative language in your shared exchanges, which may have initially seemed unlikely.

If you desire to generously cover your breasts with chocolate sauce and present them to him on a serving dish, he might respond in a profoundly sensuous manner, potentially engaging in a dialogue about the impact it had on his emotions. It is possible that she desires to apply passion fruit juice onto his physique and orally consume it. The crux of the matter is that a state of fantasy arises when one realizes that they have reached a level of profound comfort with their partner, allowing them to truly reveal themselves. That is also the point at which explicit language is initiated. Do you desire for him to don a cotton shirt during intimate moments? Some women do. Nevertheless, it is important to acknowledge that engaging in explicit language during intimate conversations must be mutually agreeable in order to be effective. Should she experience an overwhelming sensation, she might perceive an uncleanliness, although not in a desired manner. Should he lack preparedness, he may pass criticism upon her for the utterances articulated. Regardless, if both parties are unable to communicate honestly in the bedroom, the opportunity to share fantasies will remain elusive even in successful relationships. Integrity involves embracing one's true self without concealing any aspect, thereby creating an environment of tranquility.

CHAPTER TWO: NICHOLAS

DAMMIT.
That man. He was mine.
I was reluctant to even entertain the thought, however, he seemed akin to -
Like a mate.
The singular entity I had perpetually yearned for, yet perpetually eluded my grasp, notwithstanding my esteemed position as the Alpha of our pack.
The gentleman believed himself to be of human nature. I couldn't ascertain the source of my knowledge, yet it remained undeniably true. It is likely due to our connection. I'd heard stories all my life, about the miracles that could occur between mates.
Inexplicably, I possessed a certain intuition that he was a shifter,

specifically an omega, and remained oblivious to his true nature.

I failed to comprehend the feasibility of such an occurrence. However, he also harbored an attraction towards me, so we could collectively resolve the matter.

Upon successfully eliminating these coyotes.

Those infuriating creatures had returned and attempted to separate him from my possession. They had intended to compensate for that.

I felt a surge of unease as I hurriedly followed the coyotes. This inclination toward possessiveness was uncharacteristic of my usual self.

Fucking coyotes. Consistently infringing upon our jurisdiction.

The man had skillfully managed to elude their pursuit with considerable efficacy.

Following my reluctant departure from his presence, I pursued them and eventually succeeded in capturing one of them. I was usually merciful. But not today. Today, I had intended to bring about their termination. I was obliged to transmit a message.

I clamped my teeth around its fur and swiftly delivered a fatal blow to the creature's neck. If there were any positive aspects present, I would have spared its life, but it had made an attempt to harm my partner.

I carefully positioned its lifeless form upon a boulder, conspicuously exposed. I typically would have chosen to conceal it, but today is an exception. No, especially given their actions.

These coyotes were genuine creatures, without any capability to transform or change form. However, they were under the influence of mental manipulation exerted by a collective of individuals with coyote shifter abilities in the vicinity.

If the shifters were to maintain their pace, they would find themselves as the subsequent targets.

Being the sheriff of our community, it was far from desirable to be confronted with the prospect of taking the life of a shape-shifter. However, my primary identity resided in being an Alpha, and my paramount responsibility remained safeguarding our pack. My obligation to the office of the sheriff would consistently take precedence in such situations. .

I harbored a dislike towards ending a life, be it that of a creature or an animal. However, it was necessary. I had been compelled to do it previously; I had been devoid of options. It was incumbent upon me, in my capacity as the Alpha, to fulfill this responsibility. "Furthermore, no individual dared to interfere with the partner of an Alpha."

I hurriedly returned to the location where I had previously left my companion.

He wasn't there.

I sprinted swiftly, taking deep breaths, fervently seeking his scent, yet he had vanished. So was his backpack.

He had no conceivable means to depart. He was unfit to stand, let alone walk.

I conducted an exhaustive search in every possible location, yet I failed to identify any discernible evidence of any individual's footprints. I was unable to detect the aroma of anyone else either.

My heart rate rapidly increased. I'd had my mate. Presently situated directly in my view.

Subsequently, I had left him unaccompanied. And presently, his presence ceased to exist. I commenced a deliberate inquiry, methodically exploring, employing all of my faculties.

He could not be discovered within the vicinity.

How was this possible?

I observed an impression of a foot, which coincided with the precise characteristics of the boots that he was wearing. I pursued the tracks, and they persisted in leading towards the road. Then they ended.

I lowered myself to a kneeling position, observing the tracks left by the tires on the dusty surface. It appeared as though a vehicle had come to a halt. Did my associate gain access to the vehicle? Had he hitchhiked?

He may be at risk. Due to his decision to enter a vehicle, I was unable to ascertain his location. However, considering the car's previous trajectory towards the south, I would proceed in that same direction. I traversed a distance of thirty minutes behind the wheel, yet my efforts yielded no results. Just as I was on the brink of filing a report regarding a missing individual and initiating a search party, my radio suddenly came to life with a buzzing sound.

I tuned in. The radio crackled. The dispatcher said:

Trespassing with forced entry observed at the premises situated on 3525 Walton Road. The individual is a youthful male and does not exhibit signs of being in possession of any weapons. Use caution.

I grasped hold of my radio device, cordially informing them of my intention to respond to the incoming communication. I was the most suitable candidate to handle the unforeseeable calls, given that bullets, unless composed of silver, would hardly inflict any harm upon me. This fact, however, remained unknown to several of the deputies.

Once I had completed the process of infiltrating the premises, I would promptly mobilize the deputies, who possessed the ability to change forms, to initiate a search for my significant other. Subsequently, I would also retrieve the pack. I desired maximal participation from all available parties.

I personally operated a motor vehicle to the designated location. Upon arrival, I engaged in the act of cursing. That establishment belonged to a former individual known as Jimmy. It was widely recognized by all that he was extensively equipped with weapons and possessed an extensive network of surveillance cameras amounting to approximately one thousand. I accelerated swiftly, desiring to be in my jeep rather than the patrol vehicle. He was undoubtedly a source of great annoyance.

I lowered the window of my vehicle as I entered his driveway paved with gravel. From afar, I discerned the audible proclamation of Old Jimmy. I also observed his presence and held a strong belief that he brandished a firearm in a waving motion.

Adjacent to me, I briefly perceived a sight of motion. I inhaled.

Fuck. That scent!

That was my mate.

He was close. I'm curious about the reason for his close proximity to Old Jimmy. How had he arrived at this location with such haste?

It is plausible that his injuries have mended at a swifter pace than initially predicted.

I parked my vehicle at the conclusion of his driveway and swiftly exited.

I implored Jimmy to return inside the residence, cautioning that failure to comply would result in taking personal action with a firearm. He expressed discontent, yet acquiesced to my perspective, and I perceived the resonant sound of his back door shutting abruptly.

I did not wish to startle or alarm my companion. I proceeded towards the barn. I was getting closer. I could feel him.

He was sequestered in the corner of the establishment, tightly gripping a knife in one of his hands. In his opposite hand, he clasped a container filled with... peanut butter, perhaps?

Was he that hungry?

Why? The costliness of his gear indicated that he possessed sufficient financial means.

Indeed, he had sustained an injury, and his body was engaged in a recuperative process that necessitated a significantly heightened caloric intake.

However, my acquaintance was unaware of his ability to shift forms. This was bound to be intricate. I was faced with the task of conveying this information to him, but I felt it was necessary to gradually acquaint him with the concept.

I crouched down. "Hey. What is the reason for your presence in this location? Old Jimmy is crazy."

"You." He said. He pointed at me. "I saw you."

"Saw me what?"

I witnessed your transformation into a lupine creature.

Shit.

I had spent a total of twenty-eight years as a shifter, remaining undetected by any human throughout. I had received comprehensive training and remained vigilant at all times.

But he wasn't human.

I made an error in judgment due to the personal relationship I had with him. My canine companion possessed the awareness that he was in a secure state.

And...his presence perplexed my thoughts.

It was an imprudent decision on my part. He had not been prepared to witness the presence of my canine companion, not in the least. I could discern from his facial expression.

The sole advantage was that it would facilitate the disclosure of his own ancestral background now that he had witnessed my metamorphosis.

I would be compelled to simulate ignorance until I could separate him from Jimmy. There is a possibility that Jimmy may not have the capacity to cause us harm of a fatal nature, but his potential actions could significantly disrupt our well-being for a considerable period.

I would be compelled to provide false information. For now. It stood as the sole resolution. It was not feasible for me to disclose the truth to him at that moment. He was excessively near the verge of panic - I could detect its presence.

Despite the strong desire of my wolf to convey ownership to him. However, he possessed remarkable physical and intellectual prowess. It was evident from the outset that pursuing a relationship with him would pose significant challenges. "What? You saw a wolf? Where?"

He pointed at me. I did not merely perceive a wolf. I witnessed your transformation into a lupine creature."

I assumed a crouched position next to him. I experienced profound regret for my actions, however, it was necessary for me to divert his attention. "Are you feeling okay? I am aware that you are injured, but have you sustained an injury to your head?"

He cast a disapproving gaze in my direction. I did not make contact with my head. I am fully aware of what I witnessed."

Wow. He was fierce. Typically, individuals tend to falter when faced with the intense gaze of an Alpha, often without comprehending the underlying reasons behind their reaction.

But he's not human. I found it necessary to continually remind myself.

His appearance was remarkably fragile and exceptionally beautiful. I gazed upon my breathtaking partner. Despite being of average height, there was nothing ordinary about the other aspects of his appearance. His lips were plump and had a rosy hue. His complexion appeared to be supple and velvety. His nasal structure exhibited flawless alignment, just as his dental composition did.

I licked my lips. I yearned to savor his essence, yet I needed to refocus and restore our course. Allow me to pose the question to you once more. May I inquire about your presence in this vicinity?

He folded his arms across his chest and directed his gaze towards the residence of Jimmy. Attempting to distance oneself from that eccentric individual.

It appears that you entered his residence. That was crazy."

There is no necessity for him to potentially inflict harm upon me with a firearm. I provided him with a sum of five dollars."

"Five dollars?" I asked.

"Yeah. To defray the expenses incurred in acquiring the peanut butter."

Once he became under my care, I would provide him with all the necessary nourishment.

Calm down, caveman. He lacks the necessary preparedness for such a task.

I breathed in again.

His scent. He was my mate. I needed him.

Fuck. How did this unfortunate turn of events come to pass for me? Becoming infatuated with an individual of lower status in the hierarchy, who was unaware of their true nature as a supernatural being... Goodness. The group was on the verge of subjecting me to severe punishment as a result of this foolishness.

I lacked knowledge of his name. "I'm Nicholas," I said.

"I'm Avan."

Avan. I liked it. However, he still required caution. Despite humans lacking the ability to overpower him, the vicinity was teeming with numerous other shapeshifters, none of which he had the faintest inkling of.

What was the method you employed to arrive at this location? "Did you engage in hitchhiking?" I inquired.

He lifted his chin. May I inquire as to the nature of your involvement in this matter?" "May I ask why you are concerned about this?

I was not accustomed to individuals inquiring about that particular matter. All members of my cohort were aware of my status as the dominant leader. I was widely recognized among the townspeople in my capacity as the sheriff.

Providing an explanation for my actions or behavior was not typically a regular occurrence during my daily routine.

However, I was not dressed in my uniform. He lacked the means to ascertain my identity. "Tell me," I growled.

He displayed nonchalance, accompanied by a subtle gesture of eye rolling. "Yes. The individuals who halted to provide me with transportation were incredibly amiable."

"Engaging in transportation with an unfamiliar individual is not advisable." I gently massaged my face. There are various possibilities that could have occurred to him.

"Why not? I permitted your assistance in tending to my bandages despite our unfamiliarity."

I ignored that jab.

He directed his gaze towards me. May I kindly request another favor from you? Could I possibly borrow your phone in order to contact a taxi?"

He wanted to leave. I could not allow such an occurrence to take place.

I exhaled. I needed to employ innovative strategies or else face the possibility of exacerbating his displeasure. It is possible that he may not react to the dominant aspect within me. I anticipate that he would be inclined to react to the presence of the sheriff.

Please join me," I remarked, extending my hand towards him. "Get up. You're under arrest."

His jaw dropped. "Arrest? Why?"

"Breaking and entering."

I extracted my shirt sleeves from my waistband. I strongly preferred not to dress him in those, but I would do so if necessary. You are entitled to exercise your right to remain silent. Any statement you make has the potential to be utilized to your detriment within a judicial setting. You are entitled to legal representation,"

I persisted in reciting the words that I had committed to memory several years prior, as he gazed at me with an expression of sheer dread.

What age is most appropriate for the education of adolescents on matters pertaining to sexuality?

Conversations pertaining to "SEX," encompassing all related aspects, were traditionally conducted exclusively among the elderly due to the inherently sensitive nature of this topic and its associated concepts. Adolescents and individuals in their early adulthood were previously prohibited from accessing that location unless they engaged in the activity covertly within their private space.

Furthermore, it is imperative that young individuals are never subjected to the mention of the term "sex." Moreover, should they accidentally express curiosity about subjects such as childbirth, conception, genitalia, or sex, it is expected that their parents, older siblings, and members of the community would reprimand and vociferously denounce them for uttering such "sacred" words.

The American Academy of Pediatrics previously observed that even in infancy, infants demonstrate a growing awareness of their bodies by engaging in the act of stroking their genital areas while unclothed. It is important to note that such behavior primarily stems from curiosity rather than being driven by sexual motives. Hence, it is advisable for parents to offer considerate and concise replies to such queries when they are posed by those young individuals.

Sex education encompasses a comprehensive range of subjects that include human sexuality, encompassing areas such as intimate relationships, sexual anatomy, sexual reproduction, sexually transmitted diseases (STDs), sexual activities, consent, sexual orientation, abstinence, contraception, as well as reproductive rights and responsibilities.

In order to facilitate the acquisition of knowledge, develop critical thinking skills, and promote sound decision-making among children and adolescents regarding topics such as healthy relationships, responsible sexual behavior, and reproductive health, it is crucial for pediatricians, educational institutions, healthcare professionals, and parents to impart education that is both evidence-based and tailored to the developmental stage of the individual. This educational initiative has the potential to mitigate and decrease the likelihood of pregnancy, HIV transmission, and contraction of sexually transmitted infections (STIs).

When initiating the topic of sexual education to one's children, it is imperative for parents to consider several factors, commencing with the suitable age for its commencement.

Parents should take the initiative to introduce comprehensive sexual education to their children at an early age. Considering the fact that children typically commence their departure from home at this stage, whether it is for educational purposes or other activities, a time frame of two to three years proves to be the most conducive for such circumstances. To deter inappropriate conduct, it is necessary for parents to provide their children with proper education regarding the anatomical terminology of all body parts. Furthermore, it is imperative that they receive guidance from their parental figure to refrain from permitting any individual to make physical contact with them, and to promptly inform said parental figure if such contact does transpire.

In light of the visual content accessible through various media platforms, it had become imperative to impart education to children at such a tender age.

As children reach a more advanced age, such as eight years old, it is imperative for parents to adopt a heightened level of clarity and transparency on this matter. It is imperative that children develop knowledge of those fundamental truths from a young age.

Moreover, given that females around that age enter a stage of breast development, it is likely that they become more attractive to individuals in general, and especially to males.

It is unnecessary to employ monikers or illustrations when discussing matters of sexuality with a child who has attained the age of eight, regardless of their gender. This holds particularly true considering that such children are frequently exposed to an abundance of visual content through television and the Internet. Once a young girl reaches the age of eight or displays the early stages of breast development, she becomes eligible to receive education of this nature.

As a consequence of disparate tendencies among children, wherein some inquire while others abstain, a definitive approach cannot be uniformly prescribed. It is expected of parents to respond to inquiries posed by their children, and in the event that no questions are posed, parents can initiate such dialogues by acquainting their children with relevant expressions; the usage of informal monikers is unnecessary. Parents may also engage in an inquiry to ascertain their children's existing knowledge, thus serving as a valuable source of information.

Parents play a crucial role in a child's life as they are the primary individuals who come to understand and engage with them from the outset. By contrast, teachers' contributions are supplemental, as children do not spend all of their time at home, particularly those who have resumed their studies.

In order for educators to take any action, it is imperative that parents first instill their children with the core knowledge, following which any additional instruction will merely serve as a complementary enhancement to their existing understanding. It is also prudent to engage in conversations regarding sexually transmitted diseases and infections due to the potential ramifications of engaging in sexual activity.

Due to their proclivity for acquiring misinformation and adopting undesirable influences, failing to provide children with comprehensive sexual education early on might entail a burden of significant magnitude in the future. The implication is that due to the lack of moral instruction, once they separate from their parents, such as when they commence schooling, they are susceptible to receiving misleading information from others, which increases the likelihood of their belief in these fallacies.

It is necessary to impart knowledge gradually to children regarding the organs and their corresponding functions as an integral component of comprehensive sexual education, encompassing more than mere information on sex and the imperative of abstaining from it at their age.

A young individual who has not received guidance in their early years from their parents regarding the perceived impropriety of homosexuality or lesbianism would lack the necessary understanding to recognize the inappropriateness of any physical contact, whether from a person of the same or opposite sex, in specific areas.

Nevertheless, had these individuals been instructed by their parents regarding the necessity for individuals of the same gender to maintain distance, they would possess a heightened consciousness of this matter, thereby ensuring its retention within their cognitive faculties. Hence, in the event that an individual were to undertake such an action, they would potentially opt to escape or promptly contact law enforcement.

In order to mitigate the risk of children being exposed to misinformation in external environments, it is imperative for parents to assume the responsibility of educating their children within the confines of their own household.

Adolescent females often hold the misconception that engaging in sexual activity will alleviate their discomfort during menstruation. A girl of this nature was susceptible to exploitation due to her erroneous belief that it would alleviate her anguish. She will not be deceived if she is aware that sexual intercourse does not alleviate the discomfort associated with menstruation. Acquiring this knowledge will enable her to harbor doubts about any man who contradicts this information.

Females typically commence menstruation at approximately the age of 10 or 11, signaling the onset of pubescent development.

It is advisable for mothers to commence imparting knowledge to their children regarding the process of maturation and the anticipated physical transformations, inclusive of breast development and the occurrence of menstruation, as the onset of their initial menstrual cycle may come as a surprise. In such circumstances, it is advisable for parents to counsel their children to refrain from engaging in any activity that may incite them to unfasten or remove their trousers.

www.ingramcontent.com/pod-product-compliance
Lightning Source LLC
Chambersburg PA
CBHW051735020426
42333CB00014B/1318